DYSLEXIA

Chris Stanway and Lorna Miles

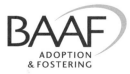

BAAF
ADOPTION
& FOSTERING

Published by
British Association for Adoption & Fostering
(BAAF)
Saffron House
6–10 Kirby Street
London EC1N 8TS
www.baaf.org.uk

Charity registration 275689 (England and Wales)
and SC039337 (Scotland)

British Library Cataloguing in Publication Data
A catalogue record for this book is available from the British Library

ISBN 978 1 907585 46 3

Project management by Jo Francis, Publications Department, BAAF
Designed and typeset by Fravashi Aga
Printed in Great Britain by the Lavenham Press

BAAF is the leading UK-wide membership organisation for all those
concerned with adoption, fostering and child care issues.

Contents

Note about the authors

Chris Stanway has worked in education all her working life. She taught in mainstream schools for over 30 years, undertaking a wide variety of roles – from the pastoral responsibilities of being a Head of Year, to curriculum and assessment management. As a SENCO (Special Educational Needs Co-ordinator), she had management responsibility for providing resources for dyslexic children. Chris developed the role of Designated Teacher for Looked After Children and worked closely with social services to set up local area networks. As a senior manager, she established and ran an inclusion unit within a mainstream school for children with a range of behavioural and emotional difficulties.

Whatever the specific job title, positive ways of working with children who were finding life and learning in school difficult has always been her strong motivation.

Together with Kate Cairns, she wrote *Learn the Child: Helping looked after children to learn*, published by BAAF in 2004. Chris now works as a training consultant.
chris.stanway@dsl.pipex.com

Lorna Miles is an adoptive parent and has been a foster carer on and off for 25 years. In addition, she has worked with children in care in a variety of settings. She is involved in training foster carers and, since the publication of *Holding on and Hanging in* by BAAF in 2010, she has been running workshops on attachment.
www.lornamiles.co.uk

The series editor

The editor of this series, **Hedi Argent**, is an established author/editor for BAAF. Her books cover a wide range of family placement topics; she has written several guides and a story book for young children.

Looking behind the label...

Jack has mild learning difficulties and displays some characteristics of ADHD and it is uncertain whether this will increase...

Beth and Mary both have a diagnosis of global developmental delay...

Abigail's birth mother has a history of substance abuse. There is no clear evidence that Abigail was prenatally exposed to drugs but her new family will have to accept some kind of developmental uncertainty...

Jade has some literacy and numeracy difficulties, but has made some improvement with the support of a learning mentor...

Prospective adopters and carers are often faced with the prospect of having to decide whether they can care for a child with a health need or condition they know little about and have no direct experience of. No easy task...

Will Jack's learning difficulties become more severe?
Will Beth and Mary be able to catch up?
When will it be clear whether or not Abigail has been affected by parental substance misuse?
And will Jade need a learning mentor throughout her school life?

It can be difficult to know where to turn for reliable information. What lies behind the diagnoses and "labels" that many looked after children bring with them? And what will it be like to live with them? How will they benefit from family life?

Parenting Matters is a unique series, "inspired" by the terms used – and the need to "decode them" – in profiles of children needing new permanent families. Each title provides expert knowledge about a particular condition, coupled with facts, figures and guidance presented in a straightforward and accessible style. Each book also describes what it is like to parent an affected child, with adopters and foster carers "telling it like it is", sharing their parenting experiences, and offering useful advice. This combination of expert information and first-hand experiences will help readers to gain understanding, and to make informed decisions.

Titles in the series will deal with a wide range of health conditions and steer readers to where they can get more information. They will offer a sound introduction to the topic under consideration and offer a glimpse of what it would be like to live with a "labelled" child. Most importantly, this series will look behind the label and give families the confidence to look more closely at a child whom they otherwise might have passed by.

Keep up with new titles as they are published by signing up to our newsletter on www.baaf.org.uk/bookshop.

Shaila Shah

Introduction

This book is concerned with dyslexia, and the particular needs of children, particularly adopted and looked after children, who have this condition.

The first half of the book starts with a short explanation of dyslexia and related conditions, including dyspraxia; their symptoms, prognosis and treatment in children and young people are outlined clearly and simply. It goes on to look at the different ways in which dyslexia can affect child development; the issues it raises with regard to educational provision for affected children, particularly adopted and looked after children, and where and how to get help.

The second half of the book tells the story of Lorna Miles and her experience of parenting a child with dyslexia, and how this affected day-to-day family life.

SECTION 1

UNDERSTANDING DYSLEXIA

CHRIS STANWAY

CHAPTER 1

What is dyslexia?

The term dyslexia covers a wide range of difficulties associated with a person's ability to decode the symbols that make up the written language. If you have never had problems with reading, then imagine yourself travelling on your own through, for example, rural Greece, Russia or China – or any country which uses a form of script foreign to you. When you get off the train, you look for signs to help you on your journey. You can see them all around you – but to you they mean nothing. It is clear that they are giving other people information, as no one else seems lost or uncertain, but the message is lost on you. Worse still, you cannot even begin to guess how to say the word, as the symbols give you no clue as to how they sound. How do you feel? A stranger in an unfriendly world? Worried? Anxious? Like someone with dyslexia?

This view of dyslexia, while being helpful in encouraging empathy with how a dyslexic person might feel, is not sufficient as a description of the condition. For the exact nature of dyslexia – the word coming from the Greek "dys", meaning difficulty with, or absence of, and "lexis", meaning words or language – has been the subject of heated debate for many years.

The word dyslexia was first used in 1887 by an ophthalmologist, Rudolf Berlin, and much early research centred around the idea of dyslexia having its root causes in sight. Indeed, it was often referred to as "word blindness". The syndrome continued to be considered as primarily a medical problem for many years. In the mid-20th century, however, the emphasis shifted to it being re-defined as an educational concern, with educational psychologists undertaking the assessments.

Dyslexia, perhaps more than any other learning difficulty, has attracted support from independent institutions and charities set up to promote research, understanding and different teaching methods for dyslexic children. In the UK, the British Dyslexia Association and Dyslexia Action have been hugely influential and provide an enormous amount of support to parents and for training specialist staff.

The following quite general definition provides some idea of the breadth of possible areas of learning affected by dyslexia, and highlights the balance between strengths and weaknesses.

Dyslexia is best described as a combination of abilities and difficulties that affect the learning process in one or more areas of reading, spelling and writing. Accompanying weaknesses may be identified in speed of processing, short-term memory, sequencing and organisation, auditory and/or visual perception, spoken language and motor skills. It is particularly related to mastering and using written language, which may include alphabetic, numeric and musical notation.

Some children have outstanding creative skills, others have strong oral skills. Some have no outstanding talents. All have strengths.

(Lindsay Peer, Education Director of the British Dyslexia Association (BDA), 2003)

However, there are opposing views about both the origins of, and best approaches towards, supporting dyslexic children. A different focus emerged following Gardner's research on multiple intelligences (2011). This book has had a significant impact on education, encouraging new ways of thinking in many areas of practice. This includes the understanding of the nature of dyslexia as it has evolved from being considered 30 years ago as some kind of deficit to today being understood as a difference.

Ongoing research into brain function provides evidence to support this perspective, as it is now possible for researchers to see where the neural connections are occurring. Non-dyslexic children use mainly the left brain hemisphere – good at processing symbols in a sequential way – for language work. But dyslexic children make many more connections to the right side of the brain. This side is primarily set up to be concerned with "whole picture thinking", which is not well adapted to accurate decoding of print. Processing from that "whole picture" down to the constituent parts takes much longer when using this hemisphere – and will certainly be much harder work!

Gavin Reid, a renowned author and consultant on the subject of dyslexia, espouses this vision (2011) and has developed the following definition:

Dyslexia is a processing difference characterised by difficulties in learning and:

- it can affect cognition, such as memory, speed of processing, time management, co-ordination and directional aspects;

- it can involve visual and phonological difficulties;

- there are usually discrepancies in performance;

- it is important that the individual differences, learning styles and work contexts are acknowledged.

Dyslexia and related conditions

This different thinking can bring many gifts of insight, creativity and originality, but there is no doubt that it also poses significant problems for the dyslexic learner. The ability to use written language is a vital skill, unlocking the way into all parts of the educational curriculum. Difficulty in learning written language is likely to impede the rest of a pupil's learning.

You may come across the term Specific Learning Difficulty (SpLD) being used alongside or instead of dyslexia. It might be helpful if this could be thought of as Specific Learning Difference rather than difficulty: "specific" because the child is functioning at least on a par with his peers except in a limited number of areas. However, the terminology SpLD may well be useful, particularly in education, as dyslexia often overlaps with a number of other conditions such as **dyspraxia** (difficulty with co-ordination of movement leading to clumsiness and problems with language), **dyscalculia** (difficulty in understanding the idea of numbers with consequent problems in acquiring numeracy skills), and **ADD/ADHD** (difficulties with maintaining focus, concentration and impulse control). Indeed, "pure" dyslexia is the exception rather than the rule, with up to

50 per cent of children with dyslexia having ADHD symptoms, and more than half the children with dyspraxia also showing clear indications of dyslexic problems. In spite of having their own labels, all these children share some essential symptoms:

- poor short-term memory;
- sequencing problems; and
- the inability to sustain focus.

However, the presentation of behavioural and learning difficulties may vary. This variety of co-existing conditions can cause challenges for communication between different professional disciplines, for while dyslexia and dyscalculia are assessed by educational psychologists, occupational therapists or physiotherapists take a lead in managing programmes for dyspraxic children, and psychiatrists diagnose and treat children with ADD/ADHD. The potential for confusion, duplication and repetition is obvious, and, I fear, too often reported.

It is estimated that there are around 375,000 children in the UK with dyslexia, with approximately 2 million people in the UK being affected.

If you have the opportunity, visit this website to watch Professor Amanda Kirby discussing just this issue: www.dystalk.com/talks/57-dyslexia-dyspraxia-amp-overlapping-learning-difficulties. She describes how parents will come to her confused because one professional diagnoses dyspraxia, another dyslexia, and a third ADHD; all, apparently, quite different. She explains how this can be related to the time at which a developmental delay is recognised – speech difficulties being noted earlier than problems with reading. However, her clear advice to a parent is to make sure that you hold in mind the overlapping picture of your child's strengths and weaknesses, so that the whole child is being considered. Seeking out your child's strengths will build his or her self-esteem and work to make sure that the environment fits the child. Once a child is assessed as being dyslexic, then his or her individual needs, whether they are in organisation, reading, spelling or memory can be identified quite specifically.

There are many schools, generally in the private sector, that are set up to provide specifically for dyslexic children, and they have been expanding in number since the 1970s. In state schools, there have been SpLD resource units within mainstream schools for over 25 years. The Dyslexia Friendly Schools Initiative has been functioning for 10 years, and schools can apply for a quality mark from the British Dyslexia Association (BDA). In addition, there has been national training for all teachers in "Assessment for Learning", which places great emphasis on teachers understanding and meeting the individual learning needs of all children.

It is possible that there has never been a time when mainstream education has been more geared up to recognising the needs of the dyslexic child — but how far this translates into practice in your locality may be a very different question.

Summary

In 2008, the Department for Children, Schools and Families (DCSF) (now the Department for Education (DfE)) commissioned a report from Sir Jim Rose on the education provision for dyslexic children and young people (2009). His headline conclusions summed up the official attitude to dyslexia today, stating that:

I   Dyslexia is identifiable as a developmental difficulty of language learning and cognition. In other words, it is now widely accepted that dyslexia exists.

10

2   Debates about its existence should give way to building professional expertise in identifying dyslexia and developing effective ways to help learners overcome its effect.

Throughout this book, I will weave a case study of a young man I have known for many years, but never had the honour to teach. The study is split into three sections.

Case study of Tom, Part 1

Tom is now 39 years old, and was born to a scientist father and academic mother. As a child in the 1970s, Tom was considered by his primary school to be a naughty boy. He was difficult to keep on task, didn't concentrate on his lessons, was often in a daydream, wouldn't sit still or listen and asked questions all the time. His teacher thought that he had learning difficulties, and needed to work harder. His mother was at a loss to understand how Tom could remember the stories she read to him word for word, yet would have temper tantrums when she tried to get him to do his reading practice. She persuaded the school to make a full assessment and Tom was diagnosed as having dyslexia. Soon after this, Tom's mother died unexpectedly in an accident. He was eight years old.

Tom's father had relied absolutely on his wife to keep the household organised, and without her presence he was unable to cope either practically or emotionally. Tom's lively and outgoing sister was a comfort, but Tom could never get anything right as far as his father was concerned. In particular, Tom's inability to get on at school was a source of constant irritation, and he was confined to his room on most evenings – not allowed out until he finished his spelling/reading/writing. This made no difference to Tom's performance, so his father, in an attempt to do the best for his difficult son, sent the boy to a private boarding school, which claimed particular expertise in supporting children with dyslexia.

Here, Tom was told that he wasn't bright enough to do any academic subjects and he would never be able to cope with taking examinations. In place of formal lessons, he was given a timetable of games and art. As he loved both these subjects, he spent a happy enough seven years there, becoming an extremely able athlete and artist. He even gained an O Level in Fine Art when he was 15. When he left school, however, Tom was unable to write or spell even monosyllabic words and had no organisational skills. He had considerable charm and was a witty companion who put considerable energy into disguising his shortcomings, and faced up to how to make a living with characteristic good spirits.

CHAPTER 2

Dyslexia: symptoms, prognosis and treatment

Dyslexia is a condition which is for life. It defines the learning style of an individual and comes with an enormously varied and unique set of symptoms. These may cause greater or lesser barriers to learning as well as providing different ways of perception, which can be of benefit to an individual. Well-documented research indicates that other members of a dyslexic child's family are also likely to be dyslexic, although in older generations this may not have had any formal recognition. It often happens when talking with a parent about their child that sudden connections will be made: 'Well, of course, his grandfather was never able to spell,' or 'I've always said she was just like my sister – always losing things and no sense of time'.

Recent studies have identified a number of genes that may predispose an individual to developing dyslexia.

(National Institute of Neurological Disorders and Stroke, www.ninds.nih.gov/disorders/dyslexia/dyslexia.htm)

Symptoms of dyslexia

There are several helpful lists of possible signs and symptoms to look out for if you are concerned that your child might be dyslexic. Such lists cannot be diagnostic or used as checklists, but can give indications of what to notice. The following information is taken from the British Dyslexia Association website (www. bdadyslexia.org.uk/).

Persisting factors

There are many persisting factors in dyslexia, which can appear from an early age. They will still be noticeable when the dyslexic child leaves school. These include:

- a family history of dyslexia/reading difficulties;

- obvious "good" and "bad" days, for no apparent reason;

- confusion between directional words, e.g. up/down, in/out;

- difficulty with sequence, e.g. coloured bead sequence, later with days of the week or numbers.

Pre–school age	
Language indicators	Non-language indicators
• Has persistent jumbled phrases, e.g. "cobbler's club" for "toddler's club"	• May have walked early but did not crawl – was a "bottom shuffler" or "tummy wriggler".
• Substitutes words, e.g. "lampshade" for "lamppost".	• Has persistent difficulties in getting dressed efficiently and putting shoes on the correct feet.
• Inability to remember the label for known objects, e.g. table, chair.	• Enjoys being read to but shows no interest in letters or words.
• Has difficulty learning nursery rhymes and rhyming words, e.g. cat, mat, sat.	• Is often accused of not listening or paying attention.
• Later than expected speech development.	• Excessive tripping, bumping into things and falling over.
	• Has difficulty with catching, kicking or throwing a ball; with hopping and/or skipping.
	• Has difficulty with clapping a simple rhythm.

SECTION 1

Primary school age	
Language indicators	Non-language indicators
• Has particular difficulty with reading and spelling.	• Has difficulty with tying shoelaces, tie, dressing.
• Puts letters and figures the wrong way round.	• Has difficulty telling left from right, order of days of the week, months of the year, etc.
• Has difficulty remembering tables, alphabet, formulae, etc.	• Surprises you because in other ways he/she is bright and alert.
• Leaves letters out of words or puts them in the wrong order.	• Has a poor sense of direction.
• Still occasionally confuses "b" and "d" and words such as "no/on".	• Has a shorter than average attention span.
• Still needs to use fingers or marks on paper to make simple calculations.	• Lacks confidence and has a poor self-image.
• Has poor concentration.	• Avoidance strategies include the following: requesting to go to the toilet, frequently changing the subject, returning to the back of the queue for help so never reaching the front.
• Has problems understanding what he/she has read.	
• Takes longer than average to do written work.	
• Has problems processing language at speed.	• Avoidance strategies at the top of Key Stage 2 become more disruptive to class with more extreme challenging behaviour.
• Is reluctant to read.	
• Tiredness after reading.	

Age 12 or over: as for primary school plus	
Language indicators	Non-language indicators
• Still reads inaccurately. • Still has difficulties in spelling. • Needs to have instructions and telephone numbers repeated. • Gets "tied up" using long words, e.g. "preliminary", "philosophical". • Confuses places, times, dates. • Has difficulty with planning and writing essays. • Has difficulty processing complex language or long series of instructions at speed.	• Has poor confidence and self-esteem. • Has areas of strength as well as weakness.

The importance of using checklists such as these with caution must be repeated – remember the character in the Jerome K Jerome novel, *Three Men in a Boat*, who read the medical dictionary and discovered that he was suffering from every ailment known to medicine, with the exception of housemaids' knee, about which lack he felt rather hurt! The suspicion that a child might be dyslexic should be based on the display of a number of symptoms over a period of time. The non-language, behavioural indicators should also be present and be inconsistent with the age

17

or stage of development of the child.

When looking at a child, you need to put all the factors together: does this child consistently produce insufficient writing? Do they always have difficulty with learning spellings? Do they have other signs such as lack of co-ordination? If they do, then it is time to talk to the school.

Trauma mimics dyslexia

There is a further factor to take into account when considering whether an adopted or long-term fostered child has characteristics of dyslexia: the effect of trauma. There is now an appreciation, supported by a wide range of research (see references), or symptoms? that confirms that children who have suffered traumatic stress injury can have significant disadvantages when it comes to learning.

> ...from early infancy through adulthood, trauma can alter the way we view ourselves, the world around us, and alter how we process information and the way we behave and respond to our environment.
> (Steele, 2002)

The effects of trauma can show themselves through many of the indicators for dyslexia given above.

Trauma is a part of the human condition. The word trauma means injury – in this context it means, specifically, injury to the brain acquired as a result of unregulated stress. We all have to cope with traumatic events in our lives – experiences that are a threat to our safety, either physically, emotionally or mentally. When these happen, stress floods our brains with hormones. This has the effect of putting a barrier between our primitive feeling brain and the thinking centres of the brain. At the moment of suffering trauma we are literally not able to think – but we can act. We can fight or run away. Once the immediate threat has gone, then we are able to manage the stress and return to a stable state. The different sections of the brain are reconnected and so we are able to think about, and begin to sort out, the feelings caused by the event. This ability to regulate stress will help repair the damage caused to the brain.

There are three events which may have been experienced by adopted and fostered children which will have caused them stress significant enough to cause injury and disrupt brain development.

Separation from their family (applies to all looked after and adopted children)
Babies and young children are completely dependent on adults for many years. Separation from the family causes great stress even if the quality of the attachment is neglectful. Attachment theory, first proposed by John Bowlby, shows how the behaviour of the adults on whom a child depends builds the internal world and brain of the child. How a child develops the ability to think, feel and act stems from the quality of the interactions between children and their adult attachment figures.

Unmet early attachment needs (applies to all looked after and adopted children)
No one is born with the ability to regulate stress, but because stress regulation is essential in order to function in society, it is one of the earliest patterns to be laid down in the first few months of life. When children do not have their attachment needs met by their attachment figure, they may be unable to regulate stress. In this case, they will overdose on chemicals that reduce the blood supply to the brain and cause more significant damage to the connections in the brain. There may be developmental impairment in many critical areas, e.g. memory, language, problem solving, higher order thinking.

Neglect or abuse (applies to some looked after and adopted children)

Some children will have been neglected or abused before being adopted or placed in long-term care. This will have resulted in overwhelming stress affecting their development. When living and working with such children, we are dealing with children who will have suffered some degree of traumatic stress in their lives. The extent to which this has affected them may be difficult to assess. We do know, however, that trauma in childhood can give rise to complex disorders, and the impact on cognitive functions can create symptoms of learning difficulties, which have much in common with the symptoms of dyslexia. Children who have been traumatised may never remember the traumatic experience, but the physiological changes can alter their development and ways of learning.

Children who have difficulty regulating stress may:

- have disrupted sleep patterns;

- have language difficulties, including finding it hard to create spoken language;

- have short-term memory difficulties;

- be unable to tolerate excitement;

- be avoidant of a wide range of activities;

- be withdrawn or spaced out;

- be disconnected from their own experience.

Having an understanding of how traumatic stress can impact upon the development of learning does not mean making assumptions about what that trauma might have been. The intervention used with traumatised children must depend upon observation and knowledge of the child as a whole, not upon a possible history.

Traumatised children need clear structures and firm boundaries, they need safety and security, they need to be enabled and encouraged to learn and they need all this to be sturdy enough to withstand the chaos of disorder.

(Cairns and Stanway, 2004)

I can think of no better starting point for thinking about appropriate strategies for living with a child with dyslexia. The term "chaos of disorder" not only describes the unregulated behaviours of a traumatised child but also gives a graphic picture of the effects on others that a dyslexic child can have.

Prognosis for children with dyslexia

With as many as one in five of the population thought to be somewhere on the dyslexic continuum, it is hardly surprising that it is difficult to produce any hard and fast predictions about the "outcomes" for a dyslexic child. In addition to the wide variety of symptoms and their relative severity, we also have the impact of the way in which they have been addressed.

The prognosis is generally good, however, for individuals whose dyslexia is identified early, who have supportive family and friends and a strong self-image, and who are involved in a proper remediation programme.

(National Institute of Neurological Disorders and Stroke, www.ninds.nih.gov/disorders/dyslexia/dyslexia.htm.)

Treatment of dyslexia

Rose's report on identifying and teaching children with dyslexia (2009) stated that:

A good indication of the severity and persistence of dyslexic difficulties can be gained by examining how the individual responds, or has responded to, well-founded intervention.

The extent of any intervention must be tailored to the needs of the individual, for no two dyslexic children will have exactly the same bundle of symptoms. All the recent work in schools is aimed at making sure that individual teachers have a better understanding of appropriate strategies to use in the classroom so that they can react quickly. Formal assessment of dyslexia can be quite lengthy, but working as if the child is dyslexic will do no harm, for the strategies are all about good teaching.

Since the understanding of dyslexia has moved away from it being regarded as a medical condition, it is strange that there should still be such an emphasis on providing a "cure". Yet the briefest of trawls through the internet will come up with any number of well-advertised "treatments", which may or may not help your child, but will certainly not be cheap!

What is clear is that with early diagnosis and skilled interventions, it is possible to help dyslexic children improve their strategies to cope with reading and writing. A harder step to take can be working with them so that they come to accept and even be proud of the different way of thinking with which they are blessed.

One of the themes that emerges when working with dyslexic people is the feeling of low self-esteem and worthlessness. There are countless examples of how people were made to feel before their dyslexia was recognised.

- They were bullied by other children and sometimes teachers, and called "stupid" or "thick".

As a child, I was called stupid and lazy. On the SAT [Standard Assessment Test] I got 159 out of 800 in math. My parents had no idea that I had a learning disability.

(Henry Winkler, actor)

The looks, the stares, the giggles...I wanted to show everybody that I could do better and also that I could read.

(Magic Johnson, basketball legend)

- They were put into bottom stream classes where the work was uninspiring and repetitive.

He told me that his teachers reported that... he was mentally slow, unsociable, and adrift forever in his foolish dreams.

(Hans Albert Einstein, on his father, Albert Einstein)

I was, on the whole, considerably discouraged by my school days. It was not pleasant to feel oneself so completely outclassed and left behind at the beginning of the race.

(Winston Churchill)

- They were ignored or picked on by teachers for not listening.

I had to train myself to focus my attention. I became very visual and learned how to create mental images in order to comprehend what I read.

(Tom Cruise, actor)

- They had schoolwork returned covered in red ink and with no idea of what to do next.

It was quite true, and I knew it and accepted it. Writing and spelling were always terribly difficult for me. My letters were without originality. I was...an extraordinarily bad speller and have remained so until this day.

(Agatha Christie)

My teachers say I'm addled...my father thought I was stupid, and I almost decided I must be a dunce.

(Thomas Edison)

Everyone is agreed that the earlier dyslexia is identified, the sooner specific interventions can be started. It is important if you notice that your child is not making the progress at school you would expect that you make contact with the school. You may find that the class teacher shares your concerns and will be able to talk to you about what is already happening to support your child's learning.

The Codes of Practice for Special Educational Needs in England and Wales, Scotland and Northern Ireland have guidelines about provision. Chapter 5 will look at this in more detail.

CHAPTER 3

Questions to ask

This chapter focuses around the case study of Tom (started in Chapter 1), which can be used to reveal problems, prompt thought and provoke suggestions.

If you were adopting or long-term fostering Tom, what information would you take from the first part of the case study? This information could be arranged under different headings:

1   symptoms;

2   support from parents/carers; and

3   treatment strategies.

Tom before age eight

Presenting symptoms

- A naughty boy

- Difficult to keep on task

- Didn't concentrate

- Often in a daydream

- Wouldn't sit still or listen

- Asked questions all the time

- Could remember the stories his mother read to him word for word

- Temper tantrums when she tried to get him to do his reading practice

Support from home

- Mother both involved, observant and informed about dyslexia

- After her death, home had a negative impact

- No evidence of bereavement being worked through

- Father had no organisational skills (possibly undiagnosed dyslexia, had "got through" by hard work?)

- Tom given negative messages, often punished but still "failed"

- Caused his father extra stress

- Boarding school seen as a positive solution for a problem child

Treatment

- Tom given clear message that although he was an academic failure he would be helped to improve in things he was good at

- Years passed without any significant attempt to help Tom improve his literacy skills

- Years passed without any significant attempt to help Tom improve his organisational abilities

- Years passed without any significant attempt to undertake any further diagnostic observations

- No celebration of achieving a good grade at O Level

- Little evidence of forward planning to ensure that Tom had skills for the workplace

Although this case study is, we hope, rooted firmly in past practice, consider the questions you would formulate and what responses you might make, given your experience and any extra knowledge you have gained about dyslexia.

You might also like to consider what safeguards are in place now that would mean a youngster like Tom would not fall through the net in the second decade of the 21st century.

Case study of Tom, Part 2

Tom left school with an exceptional ability in swimming, and an extremely well developed memory, able to soak up facts and details readily, particularly when they concerned his love of the sea or history, which always fascinated him.

Having learned to dive during holidays spent with relatives in the south of France, he became very proficient. He discovered that he was good at teaching diving skills, having endless patience in working with nervous beginners.

However, without any formal qualifications Tom had to earn his living doing whatever unskilled job he could find – chef, taxi driver, shop assistant, care worker, crewing on boats. And it was this last job which enabled him to widen his horizons and spend long periods as a diving instructor. So expert did he become that he was employed from time to time by the navy for specialist work.

In the course of his travels, Tom was often required to maintain logs and records of the work he had done. He now has two large suitcases full of such paperwork: logs which gave dates of starting but nothing more after the first barely intelligible short entries, share the space with pages of letters of recommendation from his clients. Being completely unable to organise written work, Tom has never obtained any qualifications, and relies on being hired on the strength of his great skills and undoubted ability to teach others.

After a number of years of this wandering lifestyle, Tom's father became very ill, so Tom returned home from working in Australia to nurse him, which he did for six years until his father died.

CHAPTER **4**

How dyslexia can affect child development

There are no golden rules for parenting, but if the job of all parents is to be there for their child whenever needed, this might be rather more of a challenge when living with a dyslexic child.

Christine Ostler, in the chapter 'Fussy mothers' from her book *Dyslexia: A parents' survival guide* (1999), describes how parents become very emotional about their child's education and indeed may experience high levels of 'anxiety; frustration; anger; guilt and distress'. This accords with my experience of working with a wide range of parents of children with special needs and I believe it may be explained not only by the impact of more familiar symptoms of dyslexia, but also by living with a child whose whole experience of the world is different, not only from that of other children, but probably also from the parent themselves. Coming to a theoretical recognition of the differences in cognitive processes and the resulting difficulties with reading and spelling is relatively straightforward, but coping with your child's inability to make sense of the sequences of a clock, calendar or timetable can be so fundamentally disruptive to home life as to be almost insupportable. Possibly even more disturbing is the child's increasing lack of self-esteem, which can come from the knowledge of being different and not in line with what friends of the same age are finding easy. It is no coincidence that support groups for parents, like those listed in Useful organisations at the end of this book, are becoming increasingly common!

So what can you do if you believe that your child is dyslexic? The first step is to spend time looking at the milestones of the "normal" pattern of childhood development and consider whether you are observing significant differences in your child. Could these be related to an organisational difficulty? Remember that while children develop broadly in the same sequence, the rates of progress differ substantially, and it is important to take a "whole-child" view.

Aspects of child development

In order for such observations to have clear reference points, it is helpful to be familiar with the principal aspects of child development. One of the most useful classifications to separate out different areas of development has come from the work of Vera Fahlberg (1994). Five key areas are identified:

1   Physical development

2   Emotional development

3   Cognitive development

4   Moral development

5   Social development

Physical development

This can be observed in three connected areas.

- *Gross motor development*, which is how an individual is able to change their physical position and control large groups of muscles in order to sit, stand, walk, run, and gain a sense of balance.

- *Fine motor development*, which describes the ability of an individual to use their hands in order to eat, write and draw, dress and play.

- *Sensory development*, which is how the individual is able to use all five senses.

There has been much debate about the connection between motor development and dyslexia, with Fawcett *et al* (1996) suggesting that early motor milestones may be delayed in children later shown to have dyslexia. It has been estimated that 60 per cent of individuals with dyslexia have some gross motor difficulties (Johansson *et al*, 1995), which may cause delay in independent walking. Scientific research about the significance of these links remains cautious. Viholainen *et al* (2006) warn that:

In sum, little has yet been established with regard to a connection between motor development and dyslexia.

But they do conclude that there is a:

…strong possibility that motor and language development are intertwined, so that early delay in motor development may be associated with a delay in language development.

(Viholainen *et al*, 2006)

Emotional development

The emotional development of humans is very complex, but if emotions can be understood as a mixture of feeling and the ability to think about the feeling, then development of emotions tends to begin after the end of year one. It is how we feel about the things which happen to us that allows us to make sense of the experiences. So a pre-school child can generally:

- show sympathy for others (from three years);

- show appreciation of beauty (from three–four years);

- enjoy fun and laughter (from three–four years);

- name emotions accurately (from three–four years);

- regulate own emotions (from four years).

Cognitive development

Thinking, talking, reading, writing, mathematics, art – indeed, everything we might consider to underpin the most fundamental activities of life, depends on how our cognitive abilities have developed. Babies start to make patterns of connections in the brain upon which cognitive processes are built, so that by the end of year one, true cognitive development can begin.

Some of the cognitive milestones for toddlers are:

- imitates vertical line in drawing (from 18–24 months);

- uses number words when pointing (from 18–24 months);

- completes simple jigsaw puzzle (from 24–30 months);

- has vocabulary of about ten words (from 15–18 months);

- has vocabulary of about 300 words (from 24–30 months).

Moral development

Babies are not born with any sense of right and wrong; indeed, their brains do not have the capacity for any moral sense. As with every other area of child development, it is possible to track the process by which the understanding of what is socially acceptable and the right thing to do changes over time. Thus a toddler may focus on 'Will I get into trouble?' A pre-school child may focus on rewards, while a primary school child may reach the "conventional morality" stage and be able to:

- focus on relationships;

- recognise that other people have expectations that it is right to live up to;

- value group solidarity;

- value qualities that support group solidarity, such as loyalty;

- show victim empathy – can understand the feelings of someone they have hurt.

Moral development is never fixed but depends upon circumstance. Traumatic events can alter our normal moral perspective. In extreme danger, the survival instinct can overwhelm our normal view of ourselves as selfless personalities. Children and adolescents trying out new ways of thinking about what is right or wrong can quickly revert back to more primitive stages when under pressure.

Social development

'No man is an island' is a clear statement of the human condition. We are social beings by nature, ill suited to surviving alone. Human babies will die if not claimed by an adult, and it takes many years for children and young people to learn enough skills to become independent of their families. From the youngest age, we enjoy being around other people, and much of childhood is taken up with exploring different and widening relationships.

So the pre-school child:

- understands taking turns (from three years);

- can bargain or negotiate (from three years);

- begins co-operative group play (from four years);

- enjoys group humour – silly rhymes, names, sounds (from four years).

Feeling socially isolated because of not being able to "keep up" with other children who are becoming more socially adept can add to a negative self-image at any age. However, the teenage years are likely to be a time of increased social vulnerability for the dyslexic young person. In adolescence, the peer group may hold much more sway than family, and it is a time when being the same as the rest of your friends, having the same hobbies and interests, sharing the same sense of humour, having the same attitudes to work is more important than ever. Therefore, the risk of being socially excluded because of being different matters much more keenly.

As a child develops – never in straight lines but with twists and turns, sometimes seeming to stand still in one area then leapfrogging and missing out stages altogether – they are building up their own unique identity. If all goes well, they will have a keen sense of their strengths, being very interested in what they can do. Key events: first day at school, birthday parties, learning to read, getting prizes, first night away from home, learning to swim, starting secondary school and so on, all build up resilience and confidence.

But if development is impaired in one, or more than one area, it can dramatically disrupt the building of a positive self-image.

All children ask themselves:

- Physical: how do I look, how well can I perform in sports, how strong am I?

- Emotional: how sympathetic am I, how well do I control my emotions?

- Cognitive: how good am I at school work, how do I compare with my friends?

- Moral: how trustworthy am I?

- Social: how many friends have I got?

A child builds a narrative about him or herself based on these perceptions, and perceptions of failure can induce persistent negativity.

My paintings were used week after week as examples of poor technique by an art teacher when I was 11. I was in my mid 40s before I steeled myself to enrol for a weekend painting course. I could hardly hold a brush for shaking in the first session, but then completed a number of colourfully recognisable watercolours, and have been happily painting ever since. In this one area I had an image of myself as a failure – fortunately one that didn't spill over into the rest of my life.

Dyslexic children will commonly become acutely aware of their differences across a range of areas. This builds on their sense of themselves as failures in learning, physical activity, making and keeping friends and anything to do with the need to be organised, thus producing fairly global negativity and lack of self-belief. They can become quite expert at disguising what they find most difficult to do, for even more than most children they want to be seen as "normal". Often what they cannot do is a puzzle to them. They may well understand and be able to answer questions about a topic when they hear it – but when they look down at the paper it makes no sense to them. They might know that they should have their pencil case with them, and not understand why it is so difficult to keep track of their belongings.

Parenting tasks at different stages

One of the most critical tasks for you as parents or carers is to become as knowledgeable as possible about dyslexia and its effects – and then talk to your child about it, and find strategies to explain it in age-appropriate ways. Tell them that they think differently from lots of other people and that learning some things is harder for them than it is for other children. Notice and help them to notice the many positive gifts that they have. Tell them about all the famous people who are dyslexic. Be there for them when they are exhausted by a day at school – but train them not to use their dyslexia as an excuse. If dyslexia has been diagnosed, your child may be angry and resentful, but you can play a positive part in supporting them to understand themselves better.

A few tips to consider:

- Boost morale whenever possible.

- Listen to show you understand.

- Be patient and persistent.

- Allow extra time – for everything!

- Encourage discussion of aspects of dyslexia – with the child and family.

- Acknowledge and explore things they find difficult.

- Help them to recognise and value the things they do well.

- Work closely with the school.

- Be imaginative about providing strategies to help.

- Make time for all the family.

CHAPTER 5

Education issues

The education systems within England and Wales, Scotland and Northern Ireland are different, and use different terminology. However, many of the underlying systems of how children with dyslexia or other special educational needs are supported in education are similar.

As we go to press (early 2012), the role of education in England and Wales in meeting the needs of dyslexic children is undergoing enormous changes. A Green Paper was published in March 2011, titled *Support and Aspiration: A new approach to special educational needs and disability*, which looks to change how provision for special needs is assessed. This has been through consultation and is out for trial with 31 local authorities testing out the main proposals. The 'biggest reform…in 30 years' (Department for Education, press release, March 2011) will come into force in 2014.

The existing system in schools in England and Wales, governed by the Special Education Needs Code of Practice (2001), will remain in place for the next three years, at least in those areas where trials are not taking place. This code established a "graduated approach" to defining Special Educational Needs (SEN) and involves three tiers of intervention:

- School Action
- School Action Plus
- Statement of Special Educational Need (SEN) (Statutory Assessment)

In Scotland, the terms used for these three tiers, described by Scotland's Code of Practice, are: Internal support; External support from within education; and External support – multi-agency.

In Northern Ireland, the terms used are: Stage 1; Stage 2; and Stage 3.

The kind of "actions", or interventions, which are on offer to meet the whole range of special needs in schools fall into four categories, also graduated; the concept being that increasingly powerful interventions are made available for rising levels of need.

1   Assessment, planning and review.

2   Grouping children in different ways for teaching purposes, which could be setting by ability, or in small groups.

3   Provision of additional human resources (for instance, teaching assistants).

4   Curriculum and learning resources.

This system provides a sound basis for working with children who have special educational needs, providing that it doesn't become a "straitjacket" for the child, or is seen solely as a series of hurdles to jump over. Effective learning for individuals in the classroom is an organic process, and it is crucial that teachers are able to respond quickly and with flexibility to the specific needs of every child.

The three tiers of intervention are outlined below.

School Action

School Action is the term used in England and Wales; in Scotland, it is Internal support; and in Northern Ireland, Stage 1.

When concerns are raised, from whatever source – parent, teaching assistant or teacher – then the school will gather information from all staff members who have contact with that child. This classroom-level assessment is not about one-off testing or observation, but is part of the process of teaching and learning. As parents and carers, your contribution to this process is vital. By providing clear details about your child's character and behaviour when they are at home, you can ensure that a rounded picture of your child's strengths and weaknesses as a learner is assembled.

As a result of this information, a plan of action for any extra or different support provided by staff and facilities within the school will be agreed. For the majority of children, such support will be available in the classroom and managed by the class teacher. Where all teaching staff are fully aware of the specific learning needs of your child, and have access to appropriate resources, this in-class support can provide an excellent environment in which your child can start to thrive. It is important to have realistic expectations about what will happen, and to understand that there are no quick fixes when working to support a dyslexic child.

Knowing that you are probably in for the long haul when working with the school, try to find positive ways to make direct contact with everyone involved in teaching your child. This can be tricky, especially when many people are involved, but it is a worthwhile aim. You want to be welcomed as a helpful partner in the education process rather than as being over-protective – so here are a few tips from a teacher who has known hundreds of parents in both categories.

- Make an appointment – with a focus point, e.g. completing homework.

- Find out about what has been and is being taught.

- Have a talk with your child about their lessons – and feed back the positives.

- Seek the school's observation of your child.

- Keep to a focus and have possible solutions up your sleeve.

- Ask what you can do to support your child with their homework.

- Discuss practical suggestions regarding clear instructions for homework tasks. Is school intranet available?

- Check out what help you can give. Can you write in your child's homework books? Would it be helpful for the teacher to know how long your child spent on homework?

- Agree how you will keep in touch – notes in planner, occasional phone calls.

- Leave! Seriously, agree a time limit for the meeting and leave before it is reached if possible. Think of your first contact as more like a doctor's appointment, rather than meeting a friend for coffee. The teacher will appreciate it and your good reputation will spread.

School Action Plus

School Action Plus is the term used in England and Wales; in Scotland, it is External support from within education; in Northern Ireland, it is Stage 2.

At this stage, progress should be closely monitored so that if you or the school staff feel that the first tier is not sufficient, then a further referral can be made. This could be to a range of appropriate people such as a specialist teacher, educational psychologist, speech and language therapist or other health professional. Making such a referral is generally the responsibility of the Special Educational Needs Co-ordinator (SENCO) in England, Wales and Northern Ireland (Special Educational Needs Adviser in Scotland). With the increased levels of training recommended for all teachers, there has been an increase in the number of specialist teachers with qualifications in special needs, which includes understanding and working with dyslexic children.

You should be invited to meet any professionals to whom your child is referred in order to contribute your views about what works best and what you believe should be put in place to meet the needs of your child. These consultations with services beyond the school level should provide a more detailed and specific assessment of the particular needs of a child. The recommendations arising may well include some regular time spent with a specialist outside the classroom, or more focused in-class support from a teaching assistant in specified lessons. An Individual Education Plan (IEP) (Individualised Educational Programme in Scotland; Education Plan (EP) in Northern Ireland) should be produced. This is a planning and teaching document, which is reviewed regularly and should be available to parents and all staff concerned with the child.

These should contain:

- short-term targets;
- advised teaching strategies;
- details of resources that are available;
- success criteria;
- review dates.

These plans need to be straightforward and provide clear information in ways that everyone can understand. Reviews should evaluate School Action Plus at least twice a year and more often when first set up.

Children in foster care in England and Wales must have Personal Education Plans (PEPs) as part of their care plan, and there should be consultation between the SENCO and the Designated Teacher for Looked After Children (sometimes the same individual!) to ensure that the information is coherent and correct. The Statutory Guidance about the responsibilities of designated teachers confirms that:

It is considered good practice to align the annual review of the statement with the PEP review.
(DCSF, 2009)

In Northern Ireland, Personal Education Plans were being introduced at the time of writing.

In Scotland, a Co-ordinated Support Plan is prepared by local authorities for certain children and young people with additional support needs.

The level of support that children receive at this second tier is based on what the school is able to provide from within its own budget and resources. Many dyslexic children will be able to thrive in mainstream settings once their unique differences have been identified and consistent strategies applied by all staff to meet their needs.

Provision for dyslexic pupils may include:

- Assessment and identification of the specific areas of difference: literacy, approaches to learning, motivational style and emotional and behavioural needs.

- Structured individualised learning programmes, which may well be multi-sensory and designed to address the visual symptoms, phonological symptoms, or underlying biological basis of dyslexia.

- Information and training for class/subject teachers about:
  - the child's particular patterns of learning abilities and weaknesses.
  - techniques to enable more independent and effective learning, e.g. mind maps, study skills and brain-based approaches and use of appropriate technology including word processing and specific computer-based programmes.

- Arrangements for effective school–home liaison.

Statement of Special Educational Needs (SEN) (Statutory assessment)

Statement of Special Educational Needs is the term used in England and Wales; in Scotland, it is External support – multi-agency; in Northern Ireland, it is Stage 3.

Where children's needs are such that they require ongoing support and provision above and beyond the resources of mainstream schools, then a Statutory Assessment can be set in motion. This provides a very comprehensive assessment by gathering reports from parents, teachers, an educational psychologist, health and social care professionals and others who work with, or support, the child. The local authority in England and Wales will compile a Statement of Special Educational Needs (SEN) following the completion of the Statutory Assessment. In Northern Ireland, this would be undertaken by the education board. Issuing such a Statement provides a legal guarantee by the local authority that the child's needs will be considered.

In Scotland, education authorities are required to draw up a similar document known as a Co-ordinated Support Plan (CSP) for children who have ongoing needs arising from multiple or complex factors and who need support from other services as well as education. In Scotland, Special Educational Needs (SEN) are known as Additional Support Needs (ASN).

These documents set down the assessed needs of the child and identify the resources to enable those needs to be met. These resources cover a full range of possible interventions.

- Full-time attendance at a school with specialist input.

- Full-time attendance at a mainstream school with a specially resourced provision or in a specialist unit attached. In 2010, 15,000 children across the country had such placements.

- A stated number of hours a week teaching from specialist staff.

- Modification of buildings/classroom environment.

- Number of hours of class support from teaching assistant.

- Specialised equipment, e.g. laptop, dictaphone, access to voice recognition software, coloured overlays.

- Extra time allowance in test and examination conditions.

- Differentiated curriculum offer, including possible exemption from some subjects, e.g. modern foreign languages.

There must be a full review of the Statement each year with reports requested from all the participating agencies and staff in the school.

Stumbling blocks

There is little doubt that there are examples of tensions between schools and parents of children with dyslexia. There are stories, which do seem to be becoming less frequent, of parents becoming embroiled in long drawn-out disputes about provision for their dyslexic child. In some local authorities, this centres on the difficulty of getting through the statutory assessment process in order to get a Statement, or on the lack of suitable specialist provision in the area. This most often hits the headlines at the point when the child is taken out of the state education system to be schooled at home, or sent to a private school. There are also cases of adults seeking to take action either against their former school, which failed to identify their dyslexia, thus causing them long-term disadvantage, or against their employer for failing to make "reasonable adjustments" for dyslexia when it affects their working practices.

Such difficulties are often the result of the limited resources for special educational needs provided within mainstream schools, coming up against the pressure from parents who know that their child has quite specific needs and want to get help for them. Schools may appear to be dismissive of parents' concerns, implying that they are making too much of a fuss or are being over-protective. The breakdown in communication can be difficult to manage.

Your first and most productive option is to talk to someone in the school and to build a positive relationship with the SENCO/Special Educational Needs Adviser if at all possible. If for some reason this breaks down, you should talk with the head teacher and, failing that, you can contact the SEN Governor – every governing body should have a member nominated to take a particular interest in special educational needs.

As an adoptive parent or foster carer, you can now also look for support from the Designated Teacher for Looked after Children (Designated Senior Manager in Scotland). Every maintained school has to have an identified teacher to act as a champion for, and have oversight of, all looked after children in the school. It has been acknowledged that assessment and planning for educational support for children who are looked after can be complex, partly due to the number of different professionals involved in different aspects of their care. Statutory guidance for school governing bodies in England and Wales, titled *The Role and Responsibilities of the Designated Teacher for Looked After Children*, published in 2009, gives a clear oversight of what can be expected. This document makes specific mention of the role of the designated teacher with regard to children prior to the final adoption order; these children will have both an adoption plan and a Personal Education Plan (PEP) until the final adoption order is made, when they will no longer be designated as looked after.

> *However, his or her educational, social and emotional needs will not change overnight simply as a result of the final adoption order. Schools and designated teachers will, therefore, need to be sensitive to the arrangements for supporting the educational needs of children post adoption.*
>
> (DCSF, 2009)

What will change?

So what will change in England and Wales under the proposals set out in the 2011 Green Paper, *Support and Aspiration: A new approach to special educational needs and disability*? It would be foolish to be dogmatic about what the new SEN scene will look like in 2014, since the consultation process has only recently begun. However, a look at some of the headline points may help to explain the trends – and also what might be uppermost in the minds of schools if you live in one of the "pathfinder" local authorities.

You can check the progress of the proposed legislation on the Department for Education website at www.education.gov.uk/inthenews/inthenews/a00198359/20.

Existing system under 2001 Code of Practice	Green Paper proposals for implementation 2014
Graduated categories of need: School Action, School Action Plus	One school-based category
Statutory Assessment/ Statement	Multi-disciplinary "Education, Health and Care Plan", from birth to 25. By 2014, all children who would currently have a Statement of SEN would be entitled to a new single assessment process to identify their support needs and protect their entitlement.
Budget held by local authority/ school	Possibility of personal budgets for parents of SEN children if requested, to allow choice about services that best suit the needs of their children.
Partnership between all local services advised	Strong partnership between all local services and agencies working together to help disabled children and those with SEN.
No specific role for voluntary and community sector organisations	The role of voluntary and community sector organisations and parents strengthened.

The reasoning behind these changes is open to interpretation and a matter of opinion. However, the stated aim is to give parents:

> ...more control over support for their child and family... The proposals... are intended to extend parents' influence, build their confidence in the system and minimise its adversarial nature

so:

- local authorities... (will) communicate a clear local offer for families to clarify what support is available and from whom;

- parents have the option of personalised funding by 2014 to give them greater control over their child's support, with (the help of) trained key workers;

- parents (will) have access to transparent information about the funding which supports their child's needs.

(DfE, 2011)

As there will be a crossover period between the different systems, there is an intention to streamline the present statementing procedures to cut down the length of time taken to produce a Statement. The amount of time will be reduced from 26 weeks to a maximum of 20 weeks.

CHAPTER **6**

Where and how to get help

Throughout this book, I have made reference to the British Dyslexia Association, and their website is a mine of information about the subject. However, your particular needs as an adoptive parent or foster carer may require some more specific support. You can find plenty of excellent information on the websites of BAAF (British Association for Adoption and Fostering) at www.baaf.org.uk, and Fostering Network (www.fostering.net). Contact details for these and several other organisations can be found in Useful organisations, at the end of this book.

The agency that placed your child should be able to support your request for educational support and provision as part of their post-placement service. Post-adoption support was acknowledged by adoption legislation in the UK as being crucial to the long-term viability of adoption placements. As an adopter, you are entitled to seek post-adoption support in order to consult about a range of issues, which include educational needs. The Adoption Support

Service Adviser (ASSA)/post-adoption support worker should be your first point of contact in your local authority (the placing authority in the first three years and thereafter the local authority where you live).

There are many books and articles on dyslexia and related conditions. A small number of these, including those referenced in this book, are listed in the references.

The more information you have, and the more support you can find for yourself and your family, the more likely it is that you will be able to work together to meet the challenge of your child's dyslexia.

I conclude with the final part of the case study of Tom, for consideration and discussion.

Case study of Tom, Part 3

Whilst working in a bar, Tom had met a lawyer some ten years younger than himself. She got on well with Tom's father, who considered that they were a good match and so was pleased to be at their wedding some six months before he died. Although Tom cared for his father, they never fully repaired their relationship, and he remains bitter about the education he feels his father took from him.

Tom has developed coping strategies to hide what he strongly feels is his disability. He is verbally extremely able, with an excellent vocabulary and wide interests. He has developed enough reading strategies to extract information form non-fiction sources and is able to make good guesses from context. But give Tom a task that involves writing, and he is completely hopeless. He cannot spell even the simplest words and what he writes is unintelligible even to himself. He remains unable to organise his life, often finding himself at a complete loss about how to proceed. He is, however, adept at never putting himself into a situation where he has to display his lack of writing or organisation skills in public.

The net result is that the jobs Tom has held have been manual or low-order tasks, way below his intellectual level. He has a powerful image of himself as a failure, unable to learn, easily disillusioned and with rock-bottom self-esteem. Alongside his easy-going nature and strong interests in history and politics runs a constant sense of being a man with unfulfilled ambitions.

Tom and his wife now have two children. The youngest, a boy, at 18 months doesn't sleep for more than an hour at a time, but will take "catnaps" throughout the day. He crawls quickly but makes no attempt to walk, pulling things down on top of him rather than reaching up. He is inquisitive, reacts strongly to different voices, but makes few distinct sounds himself.

Tom recognises that his son is showing some early signs of what could be dyslexic behaviour patterns, so he has enrolled in an adult literacy class. He is determined to work harder than ever to find some ways to cope more positively with his learning difficulties – so that he can provide a positive role model for Tom junior.

What better motivation could there be?

PARENTING CHILDREN AFFECTED BY DYSLEXIA

LORNA MILES

Lorna Miles is an adoptive parent and has been a foster carer on and off for 25 years. In addition, she has worked with children in care in a variety of settings. In this contribution, Lorna tells of her family's adoption of young twin boys, Malcolm and David.

'Mrs Miles had been requesting this assessment for over twelve months…'

'Much longer than that…', I thought as I eagerly scanned the educational psychologist's report for my son Malcolm, aged nine.

I had first started to be concerned that Malcolm was more than just a "bit behind" in the months leading up to him and his twin, David, joining the reception class at our local primary school. Both boys had attended a Montessori nursery school since the age of three, and whilst David had mastered the basic pre-reading and maths skills on the curriculum, Malcolm hadn't. Staff also reported that unless they guided Malcolm towards various activities and tasks he would just drift aimlessly.

At home both boys loved playing with Lego and David made some wonderful creations. Malcolm knew what he wanted to make but had no idea which bricks he needed to use or how to position them to create the model he wanted. Jigsaws posed a similar problem, usually resulting in Malcolm throwing the pieces across the room in frustration, and he often used to tear up pictures and paintings because 'they weren't right'.

But it was on a beautiful summer's day just a couple of weeks before the boys started school that I began to link these things together and to think that there was more to it than just developmental delay caused by low birth weight and illness. That day, I was keen to hang the washing out on the line as early as possible; David and Malcolm had finished their breakfast and were happily playing on the kitchen floor, but I knew that as soon as I stepped out into the garden their companionable play would be at risk of turning into conflict.

'I've got some very important jobs for you to do while I go and peg the washing out,' I said. As they were always keen to help, I instantly had their attention.

'David, you can get the tea towel and dry the things on the draining board and put them away. Malcolm, you can get the milk off the doorstep and put it in the fridge; make sure you only carry one bottle at a time. I won't be long and I want to see what a really good job you can do.'

I hurried into the garden, dealt with the washing and returned to the kitchen to see the draining board empty and David back on the floor playing with his toys. Before I could praise him for a job well done, Malcolm poked his head round the kitchen doorway from the hall.

'I've done it, come and see.' I looked into the hall. The front door was wide open and all the milk from the fridge was standing in neat rows on the doorstep! Malcolm was smiling from ear to ear and was clearly so proud of himself that I didn't have the heart to tell him he had made a mistake; I just moved the milk back into the fridge later. I was really puzzled. He knew that the milk "lived" in the fridge, so why on earth would he think I wanted it all on the doorstep? When I recounted the incident to my husband, Tim, later in the day, he found it quite amusing and concluded that Malcolm had simply misheard me, but I had a gut feeling it was more than that.

Malcolm had always been behind David in achieving developmental milestones; he was a little over three pounds when he was born, half of David's birth weight. David left hospital with his 17-year-old mother, Sandra, a few days after the twins were born, but Malcolm remained in hospital for several weeks. When Malcolm joined Sandra and David at home, Sandra struggled to cope. The relentless demands of two babies, without family support, were too much for her. As she became more and more exhausted, Sandra's temper snapped and the babies suffered both neglect and physical abuse. Numerous interventions were put in place to support her but finally, aged four

months, David and Malcolm were taken into care
and then placed with Tim and me for adoption when
they were nine months old. The arrival of twins was
more than we had dreamed of when we started the
adoption process after years of unsuccessful infertility
treatments, but our feelings of euphoria were brought
to an abrupt halt eight weeks into the placement.

Tim had been feeling unwell in the build-up to
Christmas and had taken to his bed on Boxing Day.
By the evening I was so concerned that I called
the out-of-hours medical service, who instructed
me to call an ambulance. Tim had pneumonia.

I had always felt sympathy towards Sandra, stuck in a
high-rise block with two babies, little idea of how to care
for them and no support from family or the boy's absent
father. But whatever my view had been, during the days
when Tim was in hospital and I was solely responsible
for the boys' every need, I was given a poignant glimpse
of what Sandra's world had been like. I cried with
relief when Tim was discharged from hospital on 30
December and hoped we would quickly be able to start
getting back to some semblance of normal family life.

The following day, our GP called to see how Tim
was recovering and found me not even out of my
pyjamas, as I had been up all night with Malcolm, who
just would not stop crying. He felt very hot and I
noticed that if I stood by the window cradling him,
or in a brightly lit room, his crying would escalate
and he would close his eyes. It was cheeky of me
but I asked our GP if he would mind checking him
over once he had seen Tim. His grim expression
indicated that the news he was about to deliver

wasn't good, but the words he uttered were more chilling than I had anticipated…suspected meningitis.

For the next two weeks I lived in a side room on the children's ward of our local hospital, my camp bed as close to Malcolm's cot as I could get it, grasping his tiny hand through the cot bars, whilst his life hung in the balance. He had the less serious form of viral meningitis but was still small for his age and had suffered the worst of the neglect and abuse, so was quite fragile.

Thankfully, Malcolm eventually turned the corner and started to recover. Once we were home again, he quickly started to gain weight and by the time he was two years old he was given a clean bill of health, apart from a comment about slight developmental delay.

But within weeks of the boys starting school, my concerns were growing: David was engaging well and was keen to get on with his reading and writing but Malcolm refused to engage in these activities and just wanted to play. I discussed this with his class teacher but was told not to worry, not to compare him to his twin, to bear in mind his previous illness and just allow him to develop at his own pace.

During the Easter holidays, we went to a nearby city to buy new shoes and get some other bits and pieces. The reward for good behaviour was a rare visit to McDonald's. Malcolm spotted McDonald's on our way to the shoe shop and reminded us that we would be having lunch there. When we came back down through the town, Malcolm stopped in his tracks.

'Wow, that's amazing, when we came by

earlier McDonald's was on that side and now
it's on this side, how did that happen?'

I looked at him in disbelief: he couldn't possibly think
that a building had moved from one side of the street
to the other, could he? One look at the puzzlement on
his face confirmed that he did! For about ten minutes
we walked back and forth in front of McDonald's,
with me trying to help him understand that it was us
changing direction that dictated whether McDonald's
was on our left or right. But Malcolm just didn't get it
and he spent the next few days recounting the tale of
the "magic" McDonald's to anyone who would listen.

At home, Malcolm always seemed to be in a
state of confusion: he found it hard to do any
task which involved sequencing and that included
getting dressed: pants worn on top of his trousers,
Batman-style, was a regular occurrence.

A visit from the school doctor early in the summer
term provided the opportunity for me to discuss
my concerns about Malcolm with someone from an
outside agency. She was sympathetic and arranged for
an occupational therapy assessment, which concluded
that Malcolm had co-ordination difficulties, and a
programme of daily activities to help him was drawn up.

By the end of the academic year, it was agreed by
everyone that Malcolm was significantly behind
and would benefit from remaining in the reception
class for a further year. Not only would he feel less
overshadowed by his twin, but also being one of the
more able in the class would boost his confidence.

Unfortunately, our decision was wrong. Firstly, Malcolm was very upset at being separated from his twin; and secondly, the teacher who had taught the class during his first year, and with whom he had built a good relationship, was moved to another class. He had a new inexperienced teacher who didn't understand his difficulties and was unable to give him the extra support he needed. By the end of the autumn term, his literacy skills had regressed, not progressed, and he was desperately unhappy. So we asked for him to be moved into the Year 1 class with David. He was moved and he was happier, but it made no difference to his work.

Year 2 saw little improvement in Malcolm's literacy and numeracy skills and our concerns were growing. By this time we had become so worried about his progress that we were funding extra tuition after school each day, but financially this wasn't sustainable in the longer term. I contacted a local organisation that provides independent advice to parents of children with "special needs". They advised that I should request a meeting with the educational psychologist (EP) and ask for a multi-disciplinary assessment (now known as a Statutory Assessment) so that all Malcolm's areas of difficulty could be investigated and an appropriate plan of action agreed upon. The EP refused, saying that she felt all of Malcolm's needs could be met by utilising the existing resources of the school. She concluded that he should receive ten minutes a day of individual help with one of the teaching assistants (TA).

Malcolm found these sessions very distressing; there was no consistency in the help he was offered as none of the teaching assistants had been trained to give this kind of support and they all had their own ideas about how things should be done. He was worried about how far he was falling behind and frustrated by not being able to get his thoughts and ideas down on paper. In his view, he could only be described as "thick".

Malcolm's third year in education was drawing to a close and things hadn't improved; I just didn't know what to do next. It was my sister who first suggested that Malcolm may have dyslexia. She had struggled with reading and writing throughout her school years and been labelled "lazy." She had hoped to become a vet and had been told that it was within her capabilities if only she would "knuckle down" and apply herself to getting the O Level results she needed. It wasn't until her early 20s, when her dream of veterinary college had faded into an unachievable goal and she was attending a course in horticulture, that she discovered she wasn't lazy or stupid: she was dyslexic.

She pointed out that many of Malcolm's difficulties were similar to her own.

- He was good at most subjects but had a block about English and maths.

- He was a very slow reader and often missed letters and words or jumped a line.

- He really struggled with spelling.

- He had poor handwriting and found letter formation difficult.

- He often reversed letters and numbers, for instance, 12 instead of 21, or si instead of is.

- He found it difficult to follow instructions in sequence.

- He had problems understanding what he was reading (comprehension).

- He confused left and right.

- He had little concept of time.

- He could answer questions orally but couldn't write the answer down.

- He struggled to copy things from the board.

- He lacked general organisational skills.

- He often misunderstanding the meaning of conversations.

She urged me to once again ask the EP for a Statutory Assessment.

By now I was beginning to feel like a "fussy parent". I could almost hear the class teacher groan as she saw me approaching the classroom, and the head teacher was often "busy" when I rang and asked to speak to her. The EP seemed to have a chronically full diary, and so it wasn't until Malcolm had been in Year 3 for some months that I finally got an appointment to meet with her again.

She was clearly not happy for me to be repeating my request for an assessment; in fact, she told me that I was wasting funds which could be used for children who did have a problem, but that legally she couldn't refuse my request. I said that if I was proved wrong and Malcolm didn't have any problems, I was sorry, but that if he did have a problem I had to know that I had done the best I could for him, and didn't want to find myself several years down the line feeling that I could have done more.

Over the following weeks various tests and assessments took place and I eagerly awaited the arrival of the EP's report. Part of me wanted it to confirm my suspicions about dyslexia so that Malcolm could get the help he needed. Another part of me wanted to be wrong and to have a much simpler explanation that would be easily resolved.

As I scanned the report my hopes rose: tests had shown that at age nine, his visual memory score equalled four years ten months and his auditory memory, five years six months; the list went on to reveal very specific difficulties, which in my view confirmed he was dyslexic.

However, as I continued reading my blood started to boil. I knew as soon as I read, 'Malcolm and his twin, David, are adopted and suffered emotional neglect in early infancy…' that the report was moving on to find another explanation for the poor results and that dyslexia wasn't going to be recognised. I was right: the report concluded that he was 'failing to make age-appropriate progress due to unfulfilled infantile dependency needs'. This wasn't the first time that any difficulties I had with the boys had appeared to be dismissed as an inevitable part of the package we had taken on when we adopted them…I sat and cried.

As a result of the report, Malcolm was given a Statement of Special Educational Needs which detailed a range of support he would receive in school, but none of it was to be delivered by specially trained teachers or teaching assistants, and it didn't provide him with a word processor (today it would, of course, be a laptop) or give him extra time to complete coursework. Malcolm was trapped in a world where his vivid imagination and ability to tell a fantastic story were being stifled because he just couldn't get things down on paper.

Time flew by and before we knew it the decision about which secondary school the boys should attend was upon us. I knew that the move from a small village primary school into the hustle and bustle of a large comprehensive, a much bigger site to negotiate, different teachers for each lesson and lots more homework could all add up to a "sink or swim" situation for Malcolm. David was doing well in school and we felt he would thrive wherever he went, so we opted for the school we felt would best meet Malcolm's needs. Although not the highest achieving school in the area, it was the smallest in terms of both numbers of students and the overall site. I knew by this time that getting a "diagnosis" of dyslexia and having this written into his Statement of Special Educational Needs would enable Malcolm to access not only specialist teaching but also technology and software to support his learning.

I contacted the Dyslexia Institute (now Dyslexia Action), a national charity that offers free information and advice on all aspects of dyslexia. They asked me to forward copies of Malcolm's educational "paperwork" to them and then rang me to discuss Malcolm's difficulties. They concluded that there were a number of "signposts" indicating he was dyslexic. Unfortunately, the only way to confirm this was to have specific tests which would look at Malcolm's ways of thinking, learning, and problem-solving strategies as well as his reading, spelling and maths skills. Getting this done privately would cost more than we could afford. My only option was to persuade the EP that these specific tests needed to be done.

By now my relationship with both the EP and to some extent the school was tense, to say the least, and by the time the boys moved on to secondary school, I had made no headway with getting Malcolm's dyslexia recognised. Despite this, life at secondary school got off to a good start, with the broader range of subjects on the curriculum offering more opportunities for Malcolm to excel. He was a talented musician and cast aside his violin, which he had been playing since the age of four, in favour of a bass guitar. He stayed after school as often as he could and, together with David, who was also a keen guitarist, formed a number of bands. Both boys were keen on basketball and joined the school team. But alongside these increased opportunities and greater independence, Malcolm's difficulties also became more apparent.

Although his reading and writing skills were slowly progressing, he was nowhere near the level of most of his peers. His lack of maths skills and organisational abilities were causing all kinds of problems both in and out of school. As Malcolm got older, his "difficulties" began to have more impact on day-to-day life: his short-term memory was dreadful and he could use something one minute and not have a clue where he had put it seconds later. His room was in a continuous state of chaos, and we spent hours looking for things he had misplaced. He needed a checklist to tick off items to make sure that he had everything he needed for school.

Homework was a major problem, as Malcolm just couldn't write down what he needed to do fast enough; he would leave the required books in school and had no idea when work needed to be handed in. His time management was appalling and he would spend hours on one piece of work, not realising that he had run out of time to complete other work. Following his timetable was almost impossible, partly because he never knew which day of the week it was and also because the school operated a two-week timetable whereby the subjects differed depending on whether it was Week 1 or Week 2. Malcolm was still unable to tell the time and was frequently late or in the wrong place at the wrong time and without any of the equipment he needed! Despite leaving home with everything he should have, he frequently left things on the school bus or put them down in the playground and forgot to pick them up again when he moved off.

Socially, both lads were starting to spend more time with their mates, often going into town in the evenings and at the weekends. Malcolm would often "double-book" himself and could only focus on the time the arrangements were due to start. He had no concept of needing time to get ready or how long that would take, and when David was ready and waiting to go, Malcolm was frequently not even dressed.

Money was a complete mystery to Malcolm; he couldn't do even very simple arithmetic. If he went into a shop and needed to buy more than one item, he couldn't work out if he had enough money, so to overcome this he would repeatedly go in and out of the shop buying one item at a time and counting the change in between each purchase. Needless to say, his friends got fed up and Malcolm either got left behind or came home without half the things he had intended to buy! I thought I had solved this problem when I found a calculator keyring, so that Malcolm could add up his purchases as he went along and check he had sufficient money before he got to the till. But being seen to do this was just too embarrassing and the attempt was soon abandoned.

During their second year at secondary school, the boys went on an educational trip to France, so getting to grips with foreign currency was required. We had asked for David to be in a different group as we felt that an unfair burden was being put on him to help Malcolm out and we were worried that resentment would start to grow. A member of staff was assigned to keep an eye on Malcolm and help him manage his money. Despite this, an ice-cream seller outside Notre Dame fleeced him out of £40 on the first day.

Each year at the annual review of Malcolm's Statement, I raised the dyslexia issue again. The provision was increasing but there seemed to be a barrier to actually putting the word "dyslexia" into the statement. I concluded from my research that acknowledging dyslexia would commit the local education authority to making far more resources available for Malcolm than they were currently providing, which of course would have cost implications.

Although it had started well, life at secondary school was becoming tougher and tougher, as the level of the work being set increased. By the time it came to making choices about the GCSE options for Malcolm, he was struggling across all subjects except those with a practical element, and was consequently in the lower groups. This often resulted in him being in a class with children who, for whatever reason, had no interest in education or had behavioural difficulties that demanded most of the teacher's attention. In my view, Malcolm's learning was being hindered because the teachers simply didn't have the time, the experience or the additional resources to give him the support he needed. He was working incredibly hard to achieve very little and his self-esteem was plummeting. If it hadn't been for his passion for music, which filled his free time, and around which his social life circulated, he would have been at serious risk of becoming isolated. We asked if it would be possible for him to take fewer GCSEs so that he could concentrate his efforts on doing well in a few subjects rather than being stretched across nine GCSEs and failing them all. Our request was refused.

Malcolm had seemed exhausted at the end of his first term of the two-year GCSE programme. I was counting down the days until the Christmas holidays so that he could relax and recharge his batteries. He assured me that, unlike David, he had no homework to complete and spent most of his time sleeping or playing his bass guitar. The holidays flew past and soon it was time to return to school. The day before term started, Malcolm remained asleep until lunchtime, and I finally woke him, concerned that he wouldn't sleep that night if he stayed in bed any longer. I suggested that he took a shower and I would make him something to eat. The bathroom is above the kitchen, and as I prepared a sandwich for him there was a clatter and a loud bang above me. I shot up the stairs and banged on the door. 'Malcolm, Malcolm, are you OK?' There was no response and after I had called and banged on the door a few times, I forced it open and found 15-year-old Malcolm out cold on the floor. As I knelt beside him he started to come round. He was unhurt and so I helped him back to his room, where he lay on his bed. I contacted our GP who asked me to bring him to the surgery immediately, but after examining him concluded that his blood sugar had dropped as a result of going so long without eating and sent us on our way.

The following morning both boys went off to school as usual and Malcolm seemed to have recovered completely. It was a 30-minute coach journey to school and that time had hardly passed when the school nurse rang to say that Malcolm had passed out on the coach. It had been a brief episode but the driver had taken him into school and reported it, "to be on the safe side". I went into school to collect him and on the car journey home it became apparent that he was completely stressed out about the whole school situation. Once we got home he went to his room, dived under the bed and slowly produced a whole pile of incomplete coursework and homework, together with a number of letters advising me that he was way behind and if he failed to hand in numerous assignments on the first day of term, detentions would follow. Even I felt overwhelmed by the amount of work that was outstanding and didn't have a clue how to help Malcolm get back on track. I rang the school and asked for an appointment with the Head the following day.

The Head was very supportive and sorry that I hadn't been contacted by phone to discuss the matter. She had already arranged for Malcolm to have some counselling and stress management sessions in school but she immediately backed off when I again broached the subject of reducing his workload.

An early review of Malcolm's Statement was convened and I put forward my suggestion that the number of GCSEs he was taking be reduced from nine to five, with the time which was then released being used for him to keep on top of his coursework, supported by his teaching assistant. At that time it was possible for the Head to temporarily exempt a student from part of the national curriculum for a period of up to six months to allow the local education authority to reassess a pupil's needs. The case officer from the local education authority wasn't averse to this idea but the school was adamant that it just wasn't possible. The school's main objection was based on health and safety grounds: the hours allocated for teaching assistant support did not cover all the time that would be freed up, and they felt that the new arrangement would mean that there were times during the week when Malcolm would be unsupervised, perhaps doing independent work in the library, and this just couldn't be allowed.

I was mystified: Malcolm had never been in trouble of any kind at school – in fact, he was a model pupil. They could rest assured that if he was supposed to be working in the library then that is where he would be. A six-month battle between myself, the school and the local education authority ensued. Whilst this battle continued, Malcolm's mental health was not improving and our GP became embroiled when he wrote a letter in support of my request. He hoped that 'common sense would prevail' and the reduction in the number of subjects would be agreed.

During this time, I continued to be supported by the independent organisation I had contacted several years earlier for advice on how to get the best help I could for Malcolm. Their in-depth knowledge of education law and words of encouragement when I felt in the depths of despair helped to keep me focused and finally, just as the academic year was about to draw to a close, the school agreed to my request.

The summer should have been about relaxation now that this decision had been made, but Malcolm had applied to a specialist music college for a place after his GCSEs and was frantically preparing for his audition. The school hadn't been very supportive of this plan and the Connexions adviser (a government service for school leavers) repeatedly suggested that being a full-time musician was a nice dream but that Malcolm needed to have a more achievable plan. Tim and I felt that if this was something Malcolm could excel at, we should at least give him the opportunity to try, even if it would mean living away from home from Monday to Friday.

Malcolm passed the audition with flying colours and was offered an unconditional place; the pressure was off as far as his GCSEs were concerned. This, together with the reduced workload and more time to keep on top of coursework, resulted in a smooth passage through the final year of GCSEs and Malcolm felt confident that he had achieved Grade C or above in all five subjects. He left school feeling positive about the future.

In preparation for his move to college, Malcolm was invited to one of the London universities for an assessment of his learning needs. The process was in-depth and took several hours. They took a copy of his Statement and spoke to Malcolm and myself at length. A couple of weeks later, the assessor rang:

'Mrs Miles, I'm sorry to bother you but I've studied all the paperwork and I can't see what support Malcolm has been receiving for his severe dyslexia and dyscalculia…'

I didn't know whether to laugh or cry. '…Dyslexia…you think he's dyslexic?'

'Most definitely, and he has dyscalculia, which affects numeracy; it's very severe in nature.' She went on to detail a package of support that would be put in place.

Finally, nearly ten years after I had first suggested that Malcolm might be dyslexic, it had been confirmed. My feelings were mixed. Of course I was delighted that Malcolm would at last be getting the specialist support he needed, but I was also angry that he had had to struggle for so long.

The high level of support Malcolm eventually received included a personal laptop, a programme that read back what he typed or dictated and a dictaphone for note-taking. Coursework printed on coloured paper rather than white for ease of reading, and meeting with his personal tutor once a day just to check that he was on track and keeping on top of his workload resulted in Malcolm really enjoying education for the first time in his life. He wasn't "thick" or "stupid"; perhaps, he suggested, those who had refused to recognise the problem fell into that category!

Obviously, living away from home at the age of 16 wasn't ideal, but Malcolm was passionate about his music and determined to pursue his dream. We had found a lovely family, just a short walk from the college, for him to live with during the week. They didn't interfere in his day-to-day life but were on hand if a problem arose. He was responsible for preparing his own meals, which of course caused timing issues for him; these were overcome by menu planning at the weekends, a weekly online supermarket delivery and detailed instructions of what to start cooking and when. Very slowly, he started to gain confidence and began to shop and plan for himself.

I was really worried about how he would manage the train journey twice a week as it involved a change of trains at a busy London station, and so we did a few "trial runs" to make sure he was familiar with the route. The illuminated signs which announced the forthcoming trains and their stops proved incredibly difficult for Malcolm to read because they went round so fast and he struggled to make sense of the 24-hour clock used to indicate the time. For every journey he needed to make, I wrote the final destination of the train and the time in 24 hour and analogue. This system worked well until track repairs necessitated making part of the journey by coach. Somehow, Malcolm got on the wrong coach and rang two hours after he should have been safely back in his digs to say that he was lost. By now it was 10pm on a Sunday evening, the station he had been dropped at was unmanned and he couldn't find anyone to ask. After he had searched around the station for some time, we established that he was in Weybridge, Surrey, but I had no idea how to get him back to where he was supposed to be. I rang the train company and was very helpfully told which train he needed to catch, and all the changes he would need to make, but they wouldn't tell me which platform the train left from for "health and safety" reasons. Tell him to read the travel information signs, they exasperatedly told me. I just could not get them to understand that the text moved too fast.

Should I despatch Tim to Surrey to rescue him? Despite it being a Sunday evening when the roads would be quiet, that would take at least two hours. Finally, I rang the Surrey police and explained the problem; they were fantastic and sent an officer to the station to put Malcolm on the right train. They then gave me the number of a taxi company that would meet him at the station and take him on the rest of the journey by car, providing I paid the £40 fare in advance. Finally, at 1am Malcolm was safely in his digs and I was crying with relief.

Being old enough to have a debit card had revolutionised Malcolm's experience of shopping. As long as he kept an eye on his bank account online or by getting his balance from a cash machine, he could shop without worrying that he did not have enough cash in hand. But one day he rang in a panic – his card had been refused when trying to buy a CD. We were puzzled as he was allowed a £100 overdraft, and we had only checked with him a few days earlier when he said he had £20 in the bank. He assured us that he hadn't spent any money in the meantime, so it was a mystery. I hastily transferred some funds into his account and said we would sort it out at the weekend when he came home. That weekend, the mystery was solved when he produced the slip from the cashpoint which, he said, showed he had £20 in the bank. In fact, he had only £20 of his overdraft left, and having bought some other bits and pieces during the week, purchasing the CD would have taken him over the limit. There were many other challenges over the next two years, but Malcolm finally achieved a Higher National Diploma and left the college awards ceremony with his head held high.

By now, it must be apparent that my account covers a period that goes back beyond the past 20 years, a time when perhaps difficulties such as dyslexia were little known and therefore of little relevance to those of us caring for a young person who may be dyslexic today. Sadly, in my experience as a foster carer, there are sometimes just as many barriers to obtaining the correct help for these young people today as there were then, and the challenges for those of us parenting them remain the same.

So often, the fact that the child has been or still is in care means that other causes are blamed for their poor progress. Whilst this may indeed be the case, I really struggle to understand the reluctance to assess the child to see if there is an underlying specific learning difficulty such as dyslexia. I recently sat in a meeting at the school of a ten-year-old currently in our care. 'I think Mark may be dyslexic,' I ventured. 'What makes you think that?' the Special Educational Needs Co-ordinator (SENCO) responded. I detailed all of the things I had noticed during the few weeks Mark had been with us: poor organisational skills, his struggles with writing and spelling. He couldn't do "joined-up" writing and so he printed and then laboriously went back and linked each letter together, over-writing to cover his tracks. His teacher, who was also present, said that she had no idea that he did this, though she had noted he was slow.

He found it extremely challenging to follow directions or instructions and I had made prompt cards for his getting up and going to bed routines and a checklist for his school bag to make sure he brought home everything he needed.

As a child who had just come into care, he was now entitled to 20 hours of "catch-up" tuition and the school was sure that would do the trick. I tried to pursue my request for him to be at least screened for dyslexia – this is a simple test which identifies the children who might need a more thorough test for possible dyslexia – but no one was listening. In fact, the SENCO looked me in the eye and said, 'Exactly why do you want this lad labelled?' 'So he can get the help he needs and isn't at risk of dropping out of education once he gets to secondary school,' I replied. Whilst my concerns were acknowledged, it was also noted that Mark was a bright, articulate boy, who was doing very well with his maths. It was true, he did present as a very bright lad and this is one of the difficulties with dyslexia: it occurs regardless of ethnicity, age or class and each person is differently affected by it. Most people assume that it only impacts on the person's ability to read and write and don't realise that it spills over into all aspects of the person's life and is a lifelong condition. Getting dyslexia recognised whilst the child is at school opens the doors to other provision throughout their life.

Dyslexia is now considered to be a disability, so students attending higher education can apply for a Disabled Student's Allowance to support their learning or for special arrangements to take the driving theory test. It also falls under the remit of the Disability Discrimination Act 1995/2005/Equality Act 2010. This legislation prohibits discrimination against disabled people in employment and in the provision of goods and services. Employers must make reasonable adjustment to their premises or employment arrangements if these substantially disadvantage a disabled employee, or prospective employee, compared to a non-disabled person. Malcolm has discovered to his cost that not all employers recognise this and was dismissed from a job he enjoyed just because he messed up some paperwork, although he had already told his boss he was struggling with it because of his dyslexia. Of course, the law was there to protect him, but despite the fact that he went to an industrial tribunal and won, the emotional cost of the situation was enormous.

The emotional effects of dyslexia are often overlooked. Frustration, anger and low self-esteem can manifest themselves as behaviour issues, which end up in exclusion from school and unhappiness. Working as hard as dyslexic children can to achieve the absolute minimum saps confidence and can lead to exhaustion as the young person repeatedly reads something over and over again to get to grips with it or to cover up their difficulty in front of others. I recently attended a support group for anyone who has experience of dyslexia, and one mother said, 'It's not what dyslexia does to those who have it: it's what society doesn't do for people with it.' It is sad that this is the case when, with the right teaching methods and support, children can learn to cope with and overcome dyslexia and go on to achieve their full potential.

So what can we do to help?

- Follow your gut feeling. If you think something is wrong, ask for your child to be assessed; if necessary, insist and go on insisting.

- Ask for help and support from outside agencies, e.g. IPSEA (Independent Parental Special Education Advice) or ACE (The Advisory Centre for Education). Dyslexia Action and the British Dyslexia Association both have helplines where you can find out what you and your child's rights are (see Useful organisations at the end of this book).

- If you are a foster carer, it can sometimes be difficult to know just how much input you can have in asking for help with the child's education. The Department for Education clarifies this in a helpful booklet, *Who*

*Does What: How social workers and carers can support
the education of children in care.* This is available as a free
download from www.education.gov.uk/publications/
standard/publicationDetail/Page1/LACWDWSD.

- Remember that dyslexic children are often creative;
  embrace what they are good at and allow them time
  to develop their skills. This can also provide a release
  from the stress that dyslexia causes them on a day-to-
  day basis.

- Break down tasks into smaller more manageable
  "bites" and don't give a long list of verbal instructions.
  Checklists that your child can tick off can be really
  helpful.

- Help your child to develop organisational skills by
  making full use of technology: alarms, electronic
  diaries, etc, are all perfectly acceptable tools today.

- "Clip art" can be a useful tool for producing pictorial
  reminders, for example, sticking a picture of some
  football boots on the front door when your child needs
  to remember their PE kit.

- Talk to others about dyslexia and the difficulties it
  causes: more awareness means less stigma is attached
  to admitting that a child is dyslexic.

References

Brunswick N (2009) *Dyslexia: A beginner's guide*, Oxford: One World Publications

Burden R (2005) *Dyslexia and Self-Concept: Seeking a dyslexic identity*, London: WHURR Publishers Ltd

Cairns K (2001) 'The effects of trauma on childhood learning', in Jackson S (ed) *Nobody Ever Told us School Mattered: Raising the educational attainments of children in care*, London: BAAF, pp 191–205

Cairns K and Stanway C (2004) *Learn the Child: Helping looked after children to learn*, London: BAAF

Department for Children, Schools and Families (2009) *The Role and Responsibilities of the Designated Teacher for Looked After Children: Statutory guidance for school governing bodies*,

London: DCSF, available at: www.education.gov.uk/publications/eOrderingDownload/01046-2009BKT-EN.PDF

Department for Education (2011) Green Paper: *Support and Aspiration: A new approach to special educational needs and disability*, London: DfE, available at: www.education.gov.uk/childrenandyoungpeople/sen/a0075339/sengreenpaper

Fawcett A, Nicolson R and Dean P (1996) 'Impaired performance of children with dyslexia on a range of cerebellar tasks', *Annals of Dyslexia*, 40, pp 259–283

Gardner H (2011) *Frames of Mind: The theory of multiple intelligences*, New York, NY: Basic Books

Johansson A, Forssberg H and Edvardsson M (1995) 'Children with poor reading, writing and motor skills', in Jacobson C and Lundberg I (eds) *Reading Development and Dyslexia*, Falkoping: Liber Utbildning, pp 108–113 (Swedish language)

Ostler C (1999) *Dyslexia: A parents' survival guide*, Godalming: Ammonite Books

Reid G (2011) *Dyslexia* (3rd edition), London and New York: Continuum Publishing

Reid G and Green S (2011) *100+ Ideas for Supporting Children with Dyslexia*, London and New York: Continuum Publishing

Rose J (2009) *Identifying and Teaching Children and Young People with Dyslexia*, Independent report from Sir Jim Rose, available at: www.education.gov.uk/publications/eOrderingDownload/00659-2009DOM-EN.pdf, ref: DCSF-00659-2009

Steele W (2002) 'Trauma's impact on learning and behaviour: A case for interventions in schools', *Trauma and Loss: Research and interventions*, 2:2, pp 34–47

Viholainen H, Ahonen T, Lyytinen P, Cantell M, Tolvanen A and Lyytinen H (2006) 'Early motor development and later language and reading skills in children at risk of familial dyslexia', *Developmental Medicine & Child Neurology*, 48:5, pp 367–373

Useful organisations

British Dyslexia Association

Provides advice and support to people with dyslexia and their families, as well as setting standards for professional expertise.

Unit 8, Bracknell Beeches

Old Bracknell Lane

Bracknell

RG12 7BW

Tel: 0845 251 9003

www.bdadyslexia.org.uk/

Dyslexia Action

Provides a wide range of support and services to all those who suffer from dyslexia.

Park House

Wick Road

Egham

Surrey

TW20 0HH
Tel: 01784 222300
www.dyslexiaaction.org.uk/

National Institute of Neurological Disorders and Stroke

A US organisation which conducts research on neurological disorders, including dyslexia. Their website gives information about dyslexia.
www.ninds.nih.gov/disorders/dyslexia/dyslexia.htm.)

Leadership Council on Child Abuse and Interpersonal Violence

The website includes a range of studies and research papers, mainly from the US, on the effect of childhood trauma on brain development.
www.leadershipcouncil.org/1/res/brain.html

Dyslexia Parents' Resource

A parents' resource website with a wealth of information on dyslexia symptoms and assessment, finding the right school for your child, and advice on setting up local dyslexia support groups.
www.dyslexia-parent.com/index.htm

Netmums

A parenting website giving information and advice about dyslexia and how parents can help their affected child.
www.netmums.com/support/special-needs/special-needs-focus-dyslexia

IPSEA (Independent Parental Special Education Advice)

A charity which offers free legally-based advice to parents of children with special educational needs in England and Wales.
Hunters Court
Debden Road
Saffron Walden

CB11 4AA
Tel: 01799 582030
www.ipsea.org.uk/

ACE (The Advisory Centre for Education)

Provides advice to parents/carers of children in state-funded schools who are experiencing difficulties with bullying, SEN, admissions and exclusion.

1c Aberdeen Studios
22 Highbury Grove
London
N5 2DQ
Advice line: 0808 800 5793 Monday to Thursday 10am-1pm
www.ace-ed.org.uk/

Adoption UK

A charity run by and for adopters, providing self-help information, advice, support and training on all aspects of adoption and adoptive parenting.

Linden House
55 The Green
South Bar Street
Banbury
OX16 9AB
Tel: 01295 752240
www.adoptionuk.org

British Association for Adoption and Fostering (BAAF)

Charity which provides information and advice for all those concerned with adoption, fostering and child care issues.

Saffron House
6-10 Kirby Street
London
EC1N 8TS
Tel: 020 7421 2600

www.baaf.org.uk

BAAF Northern Ireland

Botanic House
1–5 Botanic Avenue
Belfast
BT7 1JG
Tel: 028 9031 5494

BAAF Scotland

113 Rose Street
Edinburgh
EH2 3DT
Tel: 0131 226 9270

BAAF Cymru

7 Cleeve House
Lambourne Crescent
Cardiff
CF14 5GP
Tel: 029 2076 1155